WELLBOOST

At Home Workouts For Beginners

Simple Moves Big Results

This book was professionally typeset on Reedsy.
Find out more at reedsy.com

Contents

1

Chapter 1 Introduction

Welcome to your journey into the world of at-home fitness! This book is more than a collection of exercises; it's your personalized guide to building a healthier, stronger, and more confident version of yourself—right from the comfort of your own home. Whether you're new to working out or returning after a long break, this book is here to simplify fitness, motivate you, and help you take the first steps toward a consistent and rewarding workout routine.

Why I Wrote This Book

There's no shortage of fitness advice out there, but much of it can feel overwhelming, especially for beginners. Expensive gym memberships, intimidating equipment, and confusing programs often stop people before they even get started. I wanted to create a resource that removes those barriers and meets you where you are. The goal? To empower you with approachable, effective workouts and the mindset to stick with them, no matter your schedule or space.

This book was also born from personal experience. Like many, I once struggled to make fitness a habit. Time, motivation, and the convenience of staying home often held me back. But through trial and error, I discovered that simplicity and consistency are the keys to lasting results. I've compiled those lessons here to save you the struggle and make your fitness journey as straightforward and enjoyable as possible.

What You'll Find in This Book

Here's what you can expect from the chapters ahead:

Starting Strong: Building Your Fitness Foundation

Learn how to set realistic goals, stay motivated, and create a positive mindset around fitness.

No Equipment? No Problem!

Discover how to use bodyweight exercises and everyday household items to create effective workouts.

The Power of 15 Minutes

Short on time? Find quick, high-impact workouts that fit into even the busiest schedules.

Progress You Can See: Tracking Results at Home

Learn practical ways to measure your progress without fancy gadgets or gym tools.

Creating Your Home Workout Routine

Build a sustainable, personalized workout plan tailored to your needs and preferences.

Each chapter is designed to motivate, educate, and guide you through every step of your fitness journey. Whether your goal is weight loss, strength building, or simply feeling better in your body, this book will equip you with the tools and confidence to succeed.

Why This Book Will Benefit You

By the end of this book, you'll have a clear understanding of how to make fitness work for you, not the other way around. You'll have the skills to build and maintain a routine that fits your lifestyle, as well as a sense of accomplishment as you see your progress unfold. Most importantly, you'll discover that fitness isn't about perfection—it's about persistence and finding joy in the process.

This isn't just another fitness guide. It's your companion in creating a better you, one workout at a time. So, let's get started. Turn the page, take the first step, and let this book be the spark that lights your path to a healthier, happier life.

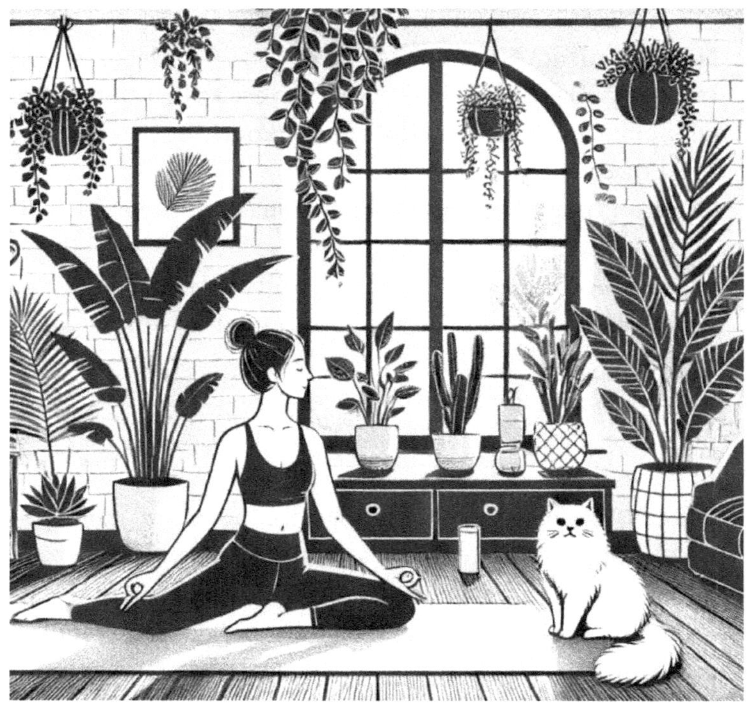

2

Chapter 2 Starting Strong: Building Your Fitness Foundation

When it comes to starting a new fitness routine, setting realistic goals is crucial for success. It helps maintain motivation and prevents disappointment when the journey doesn't meet unrealistically high expectations. To set effective goals, it's important to be specific and measurable—rather than setting a vague goal like "I want to get fit," set clear objectives such as exercising three times a week for 20 minutes each session or losing a certain amount of weight by a specific date. This level of specificity makes it easier to track progress and stay motivated as you witness the steps toward your larger goal. Starting small is also key—by beginning with manageable goals like walking for 10 minutes a day or completing a short home workout twice a week, you can build confidence and avoid feeling overwhelmed. Additionally, setting a timeframe for your goals helps maintain focus; whether it's aiming for a three-month plan to lose weight or a specific fitness milestone, a timeline provides a sense of urgency and benchmarks for progress. Finally, celebrating milestones along the way is crucial—it reinforces positive behavior and boosts motivation, making the fitness journey more enjoyable. By setting realistic, well-defined goals, you lay the groundwork for a successful fitness routine that is sustainable in the long run.

Developing the right mindset is key to achieving success in your fitness journey. It's not just about physical strength; maintaining a positive mindset can significantly impact motivation and consistency. To create the right mindset, start by focusing on your "why"—why do you want to get fit? Is it to improve your health, boost your energy levels, or feel more confident? Understanding your motivation helps in staying committed even when progress feels slow.

Visualization is a powerful tool; imagine yourself achieving your goals. This mental imagery can keep you motivated, especially on days when you feel tempted to skip a workout or fall back into unhealthy habits. Remind yourself of the progress you've already made and celebrate small wins along the way. Each workout, no matter how short or easy, is a step toward your ultimate goal.

Surround yourself with positivity—join fitness groups, follow inspiring accounts on social media, and engage with others who support your journey. Negative thoughts and self-doubt can derail progress, so practice affirmations to counteract them. Remind yourself that setbacks are part of the journey and not indicators of failure. With the right mindset, setbacks become opportunities to learn and grow stronger.

Finally, stay patient and persistent. Building a new habit takes time, and it's normal to encounter challenges. Keep a growth mindset by viewing obstacles as learning experiences rather than failures. By staying positive, keeping a clear vision of your goals, and fostering a supportive environment, you can maintain the right mindset and stay on track with your fitness journey.

To get started with exercising at home, it's essential to understand the fundamentals. This subsection will provide you with the basic knowledge needed to begin your fitness journey confidently. Start by familiarizing yourself with different types of exercises—cardio, strength training, flexibility exercises, and balance workouts. Each type plays a unique role in building a well-rounded fitness foundation.

Cardio exercises like jogging in place, jumping jacks, or high knees help improve your cardiovascular health and burn calories. These workouts are excellent for boosting your heart rate and enhancing endurance. On the other hand, strength training exercises—such as bodyweight squats, push-ups, and lunges—target specific muscle groups, helping to build strength and muscle tone. These exercises can be done without equipment, relying on your body's resistance to provide the challenge.

Incorporating flexibility exercises like yoga poses or gentle stretching routines will improve your range of motion and prevent injuries, allowing you to move more freely and comfortably. Balance exercises, such as single-leg stands or heel-to-toe walks, enhance coordination and stability, which are often overlooked but crucial for overall fitness.

Understanding these basics sets a strong foundation for your workout routine. Whether you're a beginner or just starting over, learning the core components of a balanced exercise regimen helps you build confidence and prevents overwhelm. By integrating these fundamental exercises into your home workouts, you'll be better equipped to progress effectively and safely towards your fitness goals.

Creating a solid workout routine is crucial for maintaining consistency and achieving your fitness goals. A well-structured routine combines variety and progression to keep things interesting and challenging without overwhelming you. Start by identifying your goals—do you want to lose weight, build muscle, improve endurance, or increase flexibility? The clarity of your goals will guide the structure of your routine.

Begin with short, manageable workouts—aim for sessions that last 20 to 30 minutes. This makes it easier to commit to a daily routine without feeling overwhelmed. Include a mix of exercises: cardio for heart health and fat burning, strength training to build muscle, and flexibility exercises to improve range of motion and prevent injuries. For instance, you might start with a 10-minute warm-up of jogging in place or jumping jacks, followed by 15 minutes of strength training exercises like squats, lunges, and push-ups, and finish with 5 minutes of stretching or yoga poses.

Consistency is key when building a routine. Aim to work out at the same time each day, whether it's first thing in the morning or after work. This routine helps condition your body and mind, making exercise a regular habit. To track progress, consider keeping a workout log. Record the exercises, sets, and reps, along with any notes on how you felt. This will allow you to see improvement over time and make adjustments as needed.

It's also important to listen to your body. If something feels too challenging, modify the exercise or reduce the intensity. Rest days are crucial for recovery and preventing burnout. They allow your muscles to repair and grow stronger. A well-rounded routine should include rest days—typically one or two per week—so you can continue to progress without injury.

By carefully constructing your workout routine with these principles in mind, you'll be better equipped to stick to it and achieve your fitness goals in the long run.

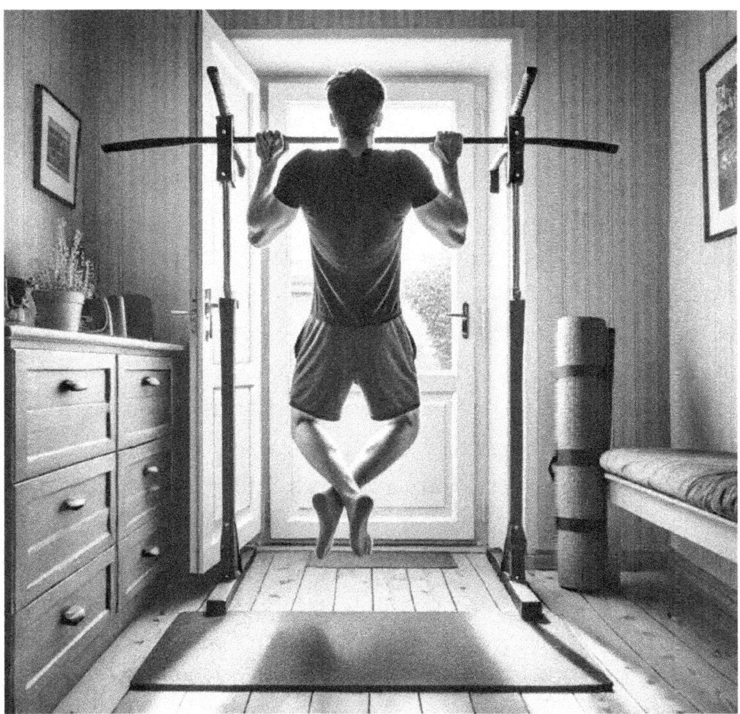

Chapter 3 No Equipment? No Problem!

No equipment workouts offer a range of benefits that make them an accessible and effective option for fitness, especially for beginners or those looking to exercise at home. These workouts rely on bodyweight exercises like squats, lunges, push-ups, and planks, which build strength, flexibility, and endurance without the need for expensive gym equipment. They also improve coordination and balance, as these exercises often require precise control and engagement of multiple muscle groups simultaneously. No equipment workouts are versatile, allowing for customization to target different fitness goals, whether it's building strength, increasing cardiovascular endurance, or enhancing flexibility. This adaptability means that individuals can progress at their own pace, gradually increasing the difficulty of exercises as their fitness level improves. Moreover, performing exercises without equipment reduces the risk of injury associated with heavy weights or machines, making these routines safer for beginners and those with limited experience in exercise. These workouts can be done anywhere—at home, outside, or even while traveling—making them convenient for anyone committed to maintaining a fitness routine regardless of their location or schedule.

No equipment workouts are incredibly versatile, making them suitable for almost anyone, anywhere, anytime. These routines can be customized to target different muscle groups, fitness levels, and goals, all while using just your body weight. Whether you're looking to build strength, increase endurance, improve flexibility, or simply stay active, no equipment workouts offer a wide range of exercises that can be adjusted in intensity and difficulty to meet individual needs. For instance, exercises like squats, lunges, and push-ups can be made more challenging by changing the tempo, adding variations (e.g., one-legged squats, clapping push-ups), or incorporating longer rest periods between sets. These workouts also allow for a full-body workout in a short amount of time, often requiring just 15-30 minutes per session. Additionally, no equipment workouts can be done in confined spaces, such as apartments or hotel rooms, making them ideal for people with busy schedules or limited access to traditional gyms. The adaptability of these exercises means you can mix and match different movements to keep the routines fresh and prevent plateaus, ensuring continued progress without the need for specialized equipment.

Functional fitness refers to exercises that mimic movements we perform in our everyday lives, emphasizing core strength, balance, and coordination. The good news is that you can achieve functional fitness without any specialized equipment by using bodyweight exercises. These exercises can improve everyday activities, such as lifting groceries, bending to tie your shoes, or reaching overhead. Examples include squats, lunges, planks, and push-ups, all of which engage multiple muscle groups simultaneously, helping to develop strength, stability, and mobility. By focusing on these movements, no equipment workouts enhance functional fitness by improving the way your body moves and performs in daily tasks. The versatility of these exercises allows for modification in intensity—whether it's the number of repetitions, rest time, or the addition of more challenging variations like single-leg exercises or explosive movements (e.g., burpees). This adaptability ensures that individuals can progress safely and continue to see results over time without needing access to a gym. No equipment functional fitness workouts can be customized to target specific areas such as strength, endurance, or mobility, making them an effective solution for those who want to stay fit and healthy without external weights or machines.

Staying motivated when you don't have access to gym equipment can be challenging, but there are effective strategies to keep your workouts engaging and enjoyable. First, set specific, achievable goals that align with your fitness level and interests.

These goals can provide a clear direction and a sense of accomplishment when you achieve them. For example, starting with simple exercises like bodyweight squats, lunges, and push-ups can build strength and confidence without the need for weights. Additionally, creating a workout playlist with your favorite music can energize your sessions, making them more enjoyable and less of a chore. Establishing a regular schedule, such as setting a specific time each day for your workouts, can help turn exercise into a habit. Incorporating variety into your routines—mixing different exercises, switching up the order, or adding high-intensity intervals—can also prevent boredom and maintain interest. Finally, finding a workout buddy or joining an online fitness community can provide support, motivation, and accountability, helping to stay committed even when exercising alone at home. By focusing on these strategies, you can make staying motivated and consistent with your no-equipment workouts more manageable and rewarding.

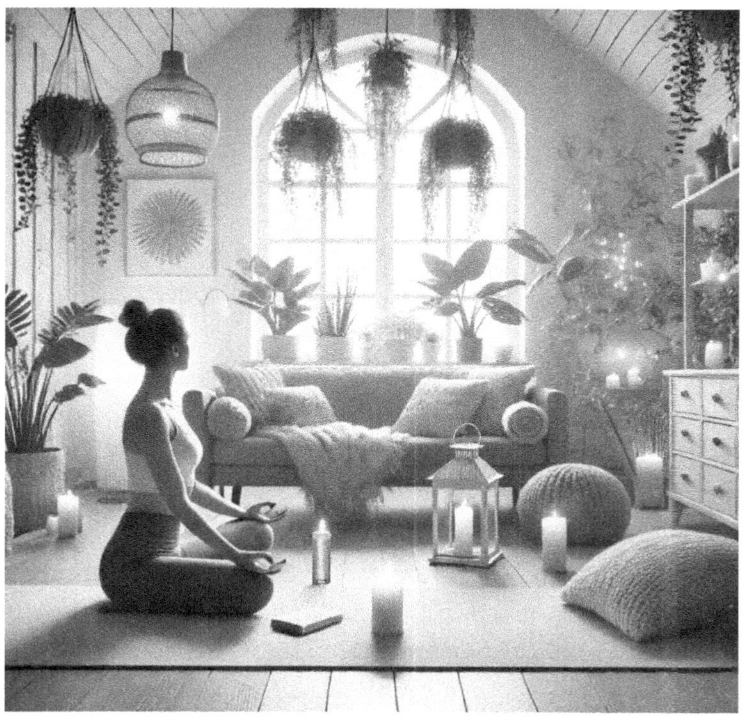

3

Chapter 4 The Power of 15 Minutes

In home workouts, 15-minute sessions can be a game-changer. By focusing on high-intensity exercises, every moment is optimized to build strength, improve endurance, and boost cardiovascular health. These short but effective sessions demonstrate that fitness isn't about the time you spend, but the quality of the effort you put in. This approach makes it easier for beginners and those with busy schedules to fit workouts into their daily routines, establishing a sustainable habit. The power of 15-minute workouts lies in their ability to provide full-body benefits, engaging multiple muscle groups and keeping the heart rate elevated for effective fat burning and fitness gains. This method not only builds physical strength but also makes exercise more accessible, manageable, and enjoyable for everyone.

Consistency is crucial in achieving and maintaining fitness gains, especially with at-home workouts. Without consistency, the effectiveness of any fitness routine can be compromised. Regularly sticking to a workout schedule, even when motivation wanes, helps build habits and routines that integrate exercise into daily life. This practice makes it easier to stay committed to a fitness regimen, despite challenges. Consistency not only leads to physical improvements—such as increased strength, better endurance, and improved flexibility—but also mental benefits, like reduced stress and enhanced mood. By making exercise a non-negotiable part of your day, you create a sustainable approach to fitness that pays off over the long term. In the end, it's not just about doing workouts occasionally; it's about the habit of consistently moving your body that will lead to real progress.

Short workouts offer a remarkable level of versatility, making them accessible to people of all fitness levels and adaptable to various goals. They can be easily modified to suit beginners, intermediate, and advanced exercisers by adjusting the intensity, duration, and types of exercises included. Short workouts can target specific muscle groups, improve cardiovascular endurance, or enhance flexibility, depending on the individual's needs. For beginners, they serve as a manageable starting point, allowing for gradual progress without overwhelming the system. More experienced individuals can use short workouts to maintain fitness or as a supplement to more intense routines. The flexibility of these workouts—whether combining high-intensity intervals with low-impact exercises, using bodyweight exercises, or incorporating bursts of activity—ensures that anyone can find a routine that fits their lifestyle and fitness objectives. By emphasizing quality over quantity, these short sessions prove that effective exercise does not always require long hours at the gym, making fitness more achievable for everyone.

Short workouts offer significant psychological benefits that can positively impact mood and mental well-being. Studies have shown that physical activity, even in short bursts, can reduce stress, anxiety, and depression by promoting the release of endorphins—often referred to as the body's natural mood lifters. Engaging in brief, intense exercises can improve focus, boost energy levels, and enhance cognitive function. Moreover, regular short workouts can help combat feelings of fatigue and boost motivation, which is crucial for maintaining a positive outlook. These quick sessions also provide a sense of accomplishment, no matter how short they are, which can improve self-esteem and reduce negative thinking patterns. By integrating these short workouts into daily routines, individuals can experience increased resilience to stress and better emotional regulation, creating a sustainable habit for long-term mental health benefits.

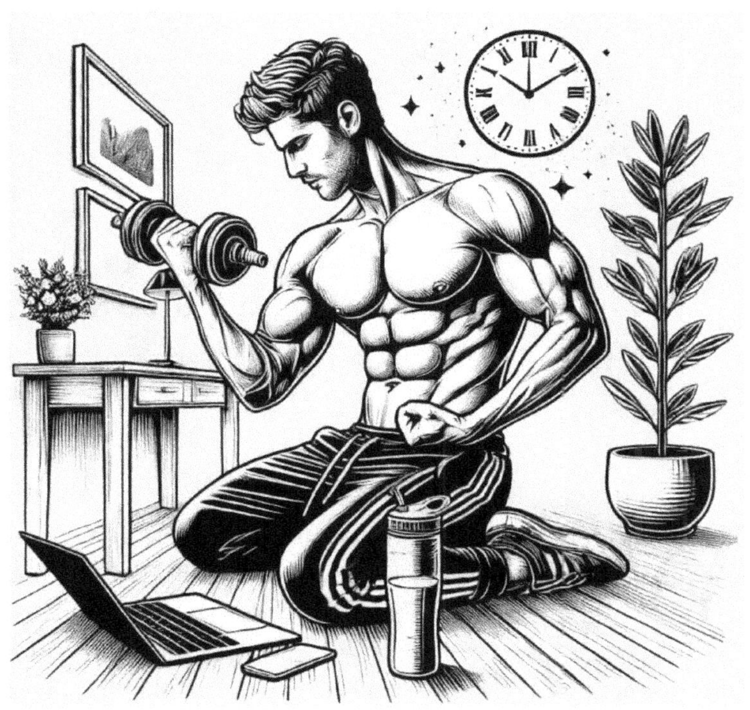

4

Chapter 5 Progress You Can See: Tracking Results at Home

When embarking on a fitness journey at home, it's crucial to set clear, realistic metrics for tracking your progress. These metrics serve as benchmarks that allow you to see where you started, monitor your improvement, and celebrate small victories along the way. Start by identifying the specific goals you want to achieve—whether it's losing weight, gaining strength, or increasing endurance.

For example, if your goal is weight loss, tracking your progress could involve measuring your weight once a week, recording the number of sets and reps you complete in workouts, or noting improvements in your exercise performance, like being able to do more push-ups or hold a plank for longer periods. If building strength is your goal, keeping track of how much weight you can lift in specific exercises can be a powerful motivator.

By establishing these clear metrics, you not only provide yourself with tangible proof of progress but also stay motivated and focused on your fitness journey. Remember, consistency in monitoring these metrics is key—whether you use a fitness app, a journal, or a simple calendar. Regularly reviewing your progress will help you adjust your routine as needed and keep you on track toward achieving your fitness goals.

When tracking your progress at home, it's essential to set realistic expectations for yourself. This not only helps in maintaining motivation but also prevents frustration that can arise from unrealistic goals. Start by acknowledging where you currently are in your fitness journey—this could involve assessing your current strength, flexibility, or endurance levels.

Setting achievable short-term goals is a good strategy. For example, instead of aiming to lose 20 pounds in a month, start with a smaller goal like losing 2-3 pounds in the first few weeks. This gradual approach makes your goals feel more manageable and gives you a sense of accomplishment as you achieve them.

It's also important to recognize that progress in fitness isn't always linear. Some weeks may be better than others, and setbacks are normal. By setting realistic expectations, you can stay committed and focused on your journey without feeling overwhelmed. This mindset allows for gradual improvements, which are sustainable and lead to long-term success.

Tracking progress at home means focusing on specific metrics that matter most to your goals. These can include measurements like weight, body fat percentage, or waist-to-hip ratio. However, it's important to look beyond the scale. Consider how your clothes fit, your energy levels throughout the day, and your ability to perform exercises that were previously challenging.

Regularly taking photos of your progress can also provide a visual representation of your hard work and changes in your physique. Seeing these transformations can be motivating and provide a more comprehensive view of your progress than numbers alone.

In addition to these physical metrics, tracking consistency in your workouts—how often you exercise, the duration of each session, and the intensity—can help you understand how your body is responding over time. By combining these approaches, you create a clear picture of your journey, allowing for adjustments as needed to continue progressing effectively.

To effectively track progress at home, it's crucial to set SMART goals—Specific, Measurable, Achievable, Relevant, and Time-bound. These types of goals help provide clear direction and structure to your fitness journey. For instance, rather than vague resolutions like "get fit" or "lose weight," aim for specific targets such as "increase my push-up count from 10 to 20 in a month" or "lose 2 inches off my waist in 6 weeks."

Setting these SMART goals allows you to monitor progress precisely and adjust your routine as needed. By focusing on detailed objectives, you can stay motivated and track the small wins that contribute to long-term success. This method of goal-setting transforms your fitness plan from a vague ambition into a strategic roadmap, fostering consistent progress and ensuring that each workout contributes meaningfully to your overall fitness journey.

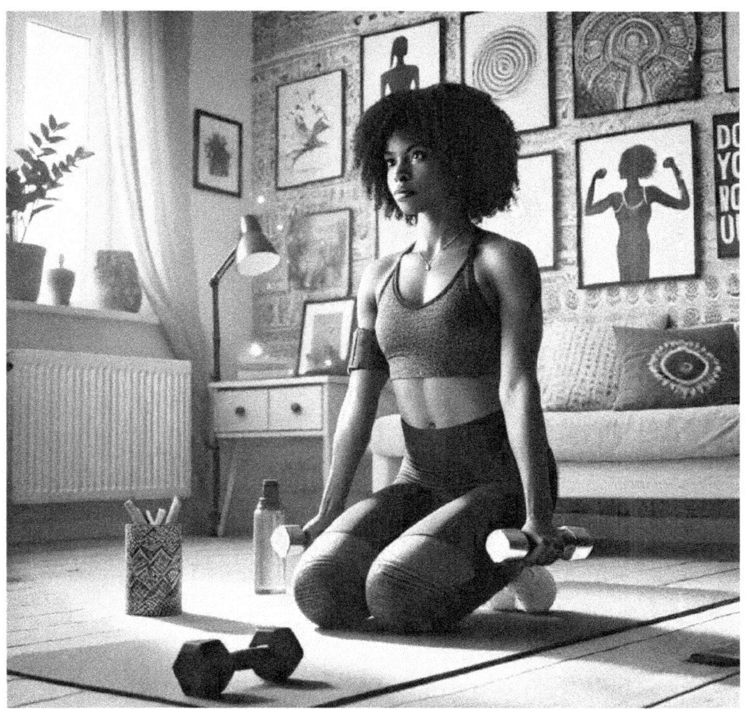

5

Chapter 6 Creating Your Home Workout Routine

Creating a consistent home workout routine starts with understanding your daily schedule and finding a specific time each day to exercise. This could be early in the morning before work, during a lunch break, or in the evening after dinner. By setting aside this dedicated time, you turn exercise into a non-negotiable part of your day, much like brushing your teeth or having a meal. This helps to form a habit that is more likely to stick in the long run. It's also important to be realistic about your availability—if your schedule is particularly busy, consider shorter, more intense workouts or multiple shorter sessions throughout the day. The key is to find a time and routine that fits your lifestyle and makes working out an achievable goal.

To build an effective home workout routine, it's crucial to design exercises that challenge your body and allow for progression over time. Start with a variety of exercises that target different muscle groups—such as squats, push-ups, planks, lunges, and burpees. By incorporating different movements, you engage various muscles and prevent plateaus. As you progress, modify the exercises to increase difficulty, such as adding weight to squats with resistance bands or adjusting the tempo of push-ups to build strength. Tracking your progress with reps, sets, or additional weights can provide motivation and keep your workouts fresh. Consistently challenging yourself is key to making noticeable progress, and it's important to celebrate small victories along the way, recognizing that gradual improvements are the foundation of long-term success.

To keep your home workout routine effective and enjoyable, it's important to incorporate flexibility and variety. This not only prevents boredom but also ensures you are continuously challenging your body in new ways. Start by including different workout modalities—such as circuit training, interval training, yoga, and pilates—so you can target various fitness aspects like strength, endurance, and flexibility. Use different types of exercises like HIIT (High-Intensity Interval Training), bodyweight exercises, and mobility drills to maintain engagement and target different muscle groups. By mixing up your routine, you also reduce the risk of overuse injuries and maintain motivation. Regularly switch between these workout types to keep things fresh and your progress consistent.

Creating a home workout routine that you can stick to requires building motivation and establishing accountability. To maintain this motivation, set clear, achievable goals—such as hitting a certain number of workouts per week or completing a specific number of repetitions. Use a workout log or an app to track your progress, celebrate your successes, and adjust your goals as needed. Join online fitness communities or find a workout buddy who shares similar goals to provide support, encouragement, and accountability. Regular check-ins with yourself or a partner can reinforce your commitment and keep you on track, even when motivation wanes. This accountability can make the difference between sticking to your routine and abandoning it when the going gets tough.

Conclusion

Completing "At Home Workouts for Beginners" marks the beginning of your journey towards a healthier, stronger you. Throughout this book, we've explored how to start from a solid foundation, the benefits of exercising without equipment, the power of short yet impactful workouts, and how to track your progress effectively. Each chapter has been designed to provide you with the tools and knowledge you need to build a sustainable routine and achieve your fitness goals from the comfort of your home.

As you move forward, remember that the key to success in fitness is consistency. By setting realistic goals, maintaining a positive mindset, and embracing the versatility of short workouts, you can make lasting changes to your strength, endurance, and overall well-being. Your commitment to regular exercise, no matter how brief, can lead to significant improvements over time. Keep challenging yourself, keep setting new milestones, and celebrate every small victory along the way.

Now that you have the guidance and strategies from this book, it's time to take action. Start today—commit to your routine, stay focused, and never underestimate the power of even a few minutes of movement. If you found value in this book, please consider sharing your experience by leaving a review on Amazon. Your feedback helps others discover this resource and encourages a community of like-minded individuals on their journey to better health. Thank you for trusting me as your guide in this journey—keep going, keep pushing, and stay strong.

Written by WellBoost

Sources: ChatGPT and OpenAI

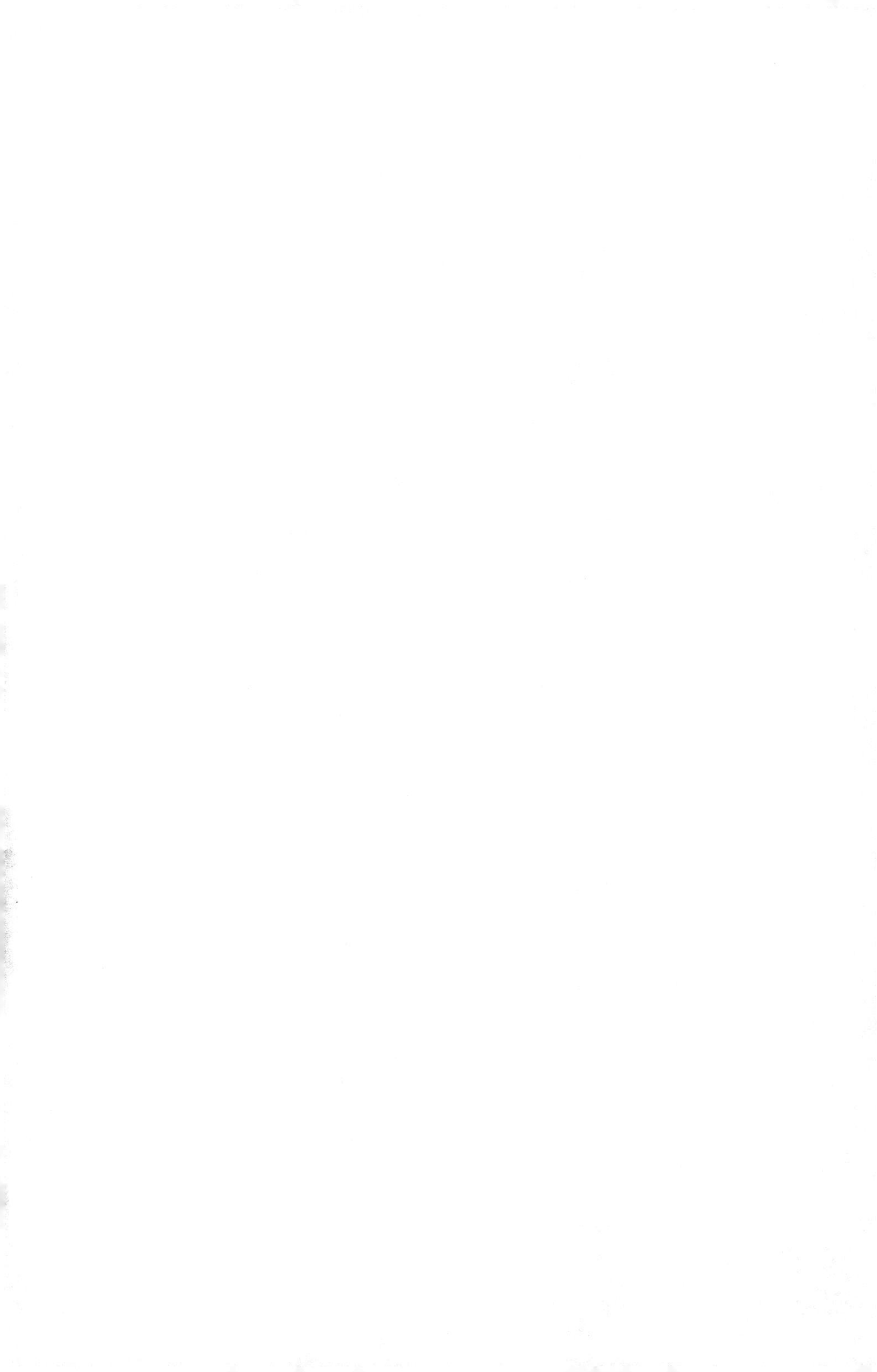